DIABETIC
COOKBOOK FOR BEGINNERS

SIMONE WILSON

Table of Contents

Introduction

Diabetes is a disease in which blood glucose, also called blood sugar, doesn't get properly regulated. Glucose is the form of sugar that's used by all cells for energy. In diabetes, the body either doesn't produce enough insulin or can't use the insulin that's produced. This a type of disease that occurs when the pancreas can't produce enough insulin, a hormone that is used to help cells use glucose (sugar) for energy. Diabetics must monitor their glucose levels regularly and take insulin to make sure the glucose stays within the normal range. Diabetes symptoms include excessive thirst, frequent urination, hunger, blurred vision, unexplained weight loss, and sudden numbness or weakness of the arms or legs. Diabetics also experienced excessive sweating, itching, and a dry mouth.

Diabetes is also a disease associated with blood sugar i.e., the concentration of sugar in the blood that the body is unable to maintain within normal limits.

Hyperglycemia occurs when blood glucose exceeds 100 mg./dl fastings or 140 mg/dl two hours after a meal. This condition may depend on a defect in function or a deficit in the production of insulin, the hormone secreted by the pancreas, used for the metabolism of sugars and other components of food to be transformed into energy for the whole organism (such as petrol for the engine).

When blood glucose levels are twice equal to or greater than 126 mg./dl, diabetes is diagnosed. High blood glucose levels—if not treated—over time, lead to chronic complications with damage to the kidneys, retina, nerves peripheral, and cardiovascular system (heart and arteries).

Causes of Diabetes and Risk Factors

Although some of the causes are completely unclear, even trivial viral infections are recognized, which can affect insulin-producing cells in the pancreas, such as:

- Measles.
- Cytomegalovirus.
- Epstein-Barr.
- Coxsackievirus.

For type 2 diabetes, however, the main risk factors are:

- Overweight and obesity.
- Genetic factors: family history increases the risk of developing type 2 diabetes.
- Ethnicity: the highest number of cases is recorded in the populations of sub-Saharan Africa and the Middle East and North Africa.
- Environmental factors are especially related to incorrect lifestyles (sedentary lifestyle and obesity).

- Gestational diabetes, which is diabetes that happens during pregnancy.
- Age: type 2 diabetes increases with increasing age, especially above the age of 65.
- Diet high in fat promotes obesity.
- Alcohol consumption.
- Sedentary lifestyle.

Signs and Symptoms of Diabetes

Symptoms of the disease, which depend on blood sugar levels, are:
- Polyuria, i.e., the high amount of urine production even during the night (nocturia).
- Polydipsia (an intense feeling of thirst).
- Polyphagia (intense hunger).
- Dry mucous membranes (the body's need to replenish fluids and severe dehydration).
- Asthenia (feeling tired).
- Weight loss.
- Frequent infections.
- Blurred vision.

In type 1 diabetes they manifest rapidly and with great intensity. In type 2 diabetes, on the other hand, symptoms are less evident, develop much slower, and may go unnoticed for months or years. Diagnosis often occurs by chance, on the occasion of tests done for any reason: the finding of a glycemia greater than 126 mg/dl allows the diagnosis of type 2 diabetes, which must be confirmed with a second dosage of glycemia and HbA1c.

Breakfast

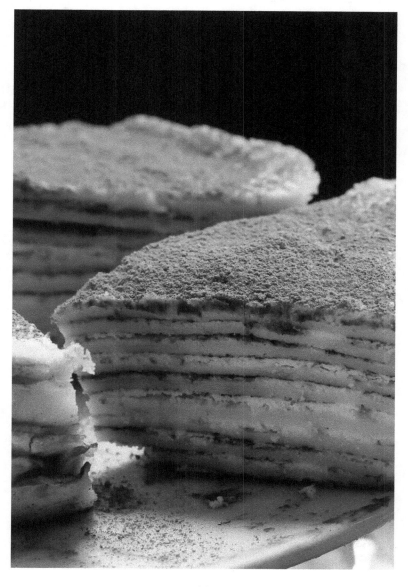

1   Crepe Cakes

Preparation time: 5 minutes | Cooking time: 20 minutes | Serves 4

Avocado oil cooking spray
4 ounces (113 g) reduced-fat plain cream cheese, softened
2 medium bananas
4 large eggs
½ teaspoon vanilla extract
⅛ teaspoon salt

1.   Heat a large skillet over low heat. Coat the cooking surface with cooking spray, and allow the pan to heat for another 2 to 3 minutes.
2.   Meanwhile, in a medium bowl, mash the cream cheese and bananas together with a fork until combined. The bananas can be a little chunky.
3.   Add the eggs, vanilla, and salt, and mix well.
4.   For each cake, drop 2 tablespoons of the batter onto the warmed skillet and use the bottom of a large spoon or ladle to spread it thin. Let it cook for 7 to 9 minutes.
5.   Flip the cake over and cook briefly, about 1 minute.

NUTRITION: calories: 175 | fat: 9g | protein: 9g | carbs: 15g | sugars: 8g | fiber: 2g | sodium: 213mg

2 Zucchini Bread

Preparation time: 15 minutes | Cooking time: 45 minutes | Serves 24

1½ cups gluten-free all-purpose flour
1 cup almond meal
½ cup chickpea flour
1 teaspoon salt
1 teaspoon baking powder
1 teaspoon baking soda
½ teaspoon ground nutmeg
½ teaspoon ground cinnamon
3 medium brown eggs
¼ cup sunflower seed oil
2 ripe bananas, mashed
2 zucchini, grated, with water squeezed out
2 teaspoons almond extract

1. Preheat the oven to 350°F (180°C). Line a 9 × 13-inch pan with parchment paper.
2. In a large bowl, use a fork or whisk to combine the gluten-free flour, almond meal, chickpea flour, salt, baking powder, baking soda, nutmeg, and cinnamon.
3. In a separate large bowl, beat the eggs, oil, bananas, zucchini, and almond extract together well.

4. Fold the dry ingredients into the wet ingredients, stir until well combined, and pour into the prepared pan.

5. Transfer the pan to the oven, and bake for 40 to 45 minutes, or until a butter knife inserted into the center comes out clean. Remove from the oven, and let the bread rest for 15 minutes before serving.

NUTRITION: calories: 203 | fat: 11g | protein: 6g | carbs: 21g | sugars: 4g | fiber: 4g | sodium: 323mg

3 Apple Filled Swedish Pancake

Prep time: 25 minutes | Cook time: 20 minutes | Serves: 6

2 apples, cored and sliced thin
¾ cup egg substitute
½ cup fat-free milk
½ cup sugar-free caramel sauce
1 tbsp. reduced calorie margarine
What you'll need from the store cupboard
½ cup flour
1 `1/2 tbsp. brown sugar substitute
2 tsp water
¼ tsp cinnamon
1/8 tsp cloves
1/8 tsp salt
Nonstick cooking spray

1.   Heat oven to 400 degrees. Place margarine in cast iron, or ovenproof, skillet and place in oven until margarine is melted.
2.   In a medium bowl, whisk together flour, milk, egg substitute, cinnamon, cloves and salt until smooth.
3.   Pour batter in hot skillet and bake 20 – 25 minutes until puffed and golden brown.

4.   Spray a medium saucepan with cooking spray. Heat over medium heat.

5.   Add apples, brown sugar and water. Cook, stirring occasionally, until apples are tender and golden brown, about 4 – 6 minutes.

6.   Pour the caramel sauce into a microwave-proof measuring glass and heat 30 – 45 seconds, or until warmed through.

7.   To serve, spoon apples into pancake and drizzle with caramel. Cut into wedges.

NUTRITION: Calories 193 Total Carbs 25g Net Carbs 23g Protein 6g Fat 2g Sugar 12g Fiber 2g

4   Cinnamon Walnut Granola

Preparation time: 10 minutes | Cooking time: 30 minutes | Serves 16

4 cups rolled oats
1 cup walnut pieces
½ cup pepitas
¼ teaspoon salt
1 teaspoon ground cinnamon
1 teaspoon ground ginger
½ cup coconut oil, melted
½ cup unsweetened applesauce
1 teaspoon vanilla extract
½ cup dried cherries

1.   Preheat the oven to 350°F (180°C). Line a baking sheet with parchment paper.
2.   In a large bowl, toss the oats, walnuts, pepitas, salt, cinnamon, and ginger.
3.   In a large measuring cup, combine the coconut oil, applesauce, and vanilla. Pour over the dry mixture and mix well.
4.   Transfer the mixture to the prepared baking sheet. Cook for 30 minutes, stirring about halfway through. Remove from the oven and let the granola sit undisturbed until completely cool. Break the granola into pieces, and stir in the dried cherries.

5.   Transfer to an airtight container, and store at room temperature for up to 2 weeks.

NUTRITION: calories: 224 | fat: 15g | protein: 5g | carbs: 20g | sugars: 5g | fiber: 3g | sodium: 30mg

5   Apple Cinnamon Scones

Prep time: 5 minutes | Cook time: 25 minutes | Serves: 16

2 large eggs
1 apple, diced
¼ cup + ½ tbsp. margarine, melted and divided
1 tbsp. half-n-half
What you'll need from store cupboard:
3 cups almond flour
1/3 cup + 2 tsp Splenda
2 tsp baking powder
2 tsp cinnamon
1 tsp vanilla
¼ tsp salt

1.   Heat oven to 325 degrees. Line a large baking sheet with parchment paper.
2.   In a large bowl, whisk flour, 1/3 cup Splenda, baking powder, 1 ½ teaspoons cinnamon, and salt together. Stir in apple.
3.   Add the eggs, ¼ cup melted margarine, cream, and vanilla. Stir until the mixture forms a soft dough.
4.   Divide the dough in half and pat into 2 circles, about 1-inch thick, and 7-8 inches around.
5.   In a small bowl, stir together remaining 2 teaspoons Splenda, and ½ teaspoon cinnamon.

6.   Brush the ½ tablespoon melted margarine over dough and sprinkle with cinnamon mixture. Cut each into 8 equal pieces and place on prepared baking sheet.

7.   Bake 20-25 minutes, or until golden brown and firm to the touch.

NUTRITION: Calories 176 Total Carbs 12g Net Carbs 9g Protein 5g Fat 12g Sugar 8g Fiber 3g

Prep time: 15 min | Cooking Time: 25 Minutes
Servings: 12 |

2 cups fresh raspberries or blueberries
2 tablespoons sugar
2 tablespoons freshly squeezed lemon juice
1 tablespoon cornstarch
11/2 cups rolled oats
1/2 cup whole-wheat flour
1/2 cup walnuts
¼ cup chia seeds
¼ cup extra-virgin olive oil
¼ cup honey
large egg

Direction:
1. Preheat the oven to 350F. In a small saucepan over medium heat, stir together the berries, sugar, lemon juice, and cornstarch.
2. Bring to a simmer. Reduce the heat and simmer for 2 to 3 minutes, until the mixture thickens.
3. In a food processor or high-speed blender, combine the oats, flour, walnuts, and chia seeds.
4. Process until powdered. Add the olive oil, honey, and egg.

5. Pulse a few more times, until well combined. Press half of the mixture into a 9-inch square baking dish. Spread the berry filling over the oat mixture. Add the remaining oat mixture on top of the berries.
6. Bake for 25 minutes, until browned. Let cool completely, cut into 12 pieces, and serve. Store in a covered container for up to 5 days.

NUTRITION: Calories: 201; Total fat: 10g; Saturated fat: 1g; Protein: 5g; Carbs: 26g; Sugar: 9g; Fiber: 5g; Sodium: 8mg

7   Eggplant Omelet

Servings: 2 Cooking Time: 5 Minutes

large eggplant
1 tbsp coconut oil, melted
1 tsp unsalted butter
2 eggs
2 tbsp chopped green onions

Direction:
1. Set the grill and let it preheat at the high setting.
2. In the meantime, prepare the eggplant, and for this, cut two slices from eggplant, about 1-inch thick, and reserve the remaining eggplant for later use.
3. Brush slices of eggplant with oil, season with salt on both sides, then put the slices on grill and cook for 3 to 4 minutes per side.
4. Move grilled eggplant to a cutting board, let it cool for 5 minutes and then make a home in the center of each slice by using a cookie cutter.
5. Bring out a frying pan, put it over medium heat, add butter and when it melts, add eggplant slices in it and crack an egg into its each hole.
6. Let the eggs cook, then carefully flip the eggplant slice and continue cooking for 3 minutes until the egg has thoroughly cooked Season egg with salt and

black pepper, move them to a plate, then garnish with green onions and serve.

NUTRITION: 184 Cal 14.1 g Fats 7.8 g Protein 3 g Net Carb 3.5 g Fiber

8   Eggs & Cocotte on Toast

Preparation Time: 10 minutes | Cooking Time: 15 minutes | Servings: 2

1/8 teaspoon of black pepper
¼ teaspoon salt
½ teaspoon Italian seasoning
¼ teaspoon balsamic vinegar
¼ teaspoon sugar-free maple syrup
1 cup sausages, chopped into small pieces
2 eggs
2 slices of whole-wheat toast
3 tablespoons cheddar cheese, shredded
6-slices tomatoes
Cooking spray
A little mayonnaise to serve

1.   Spray baking dish with cooking spray. Abode the bread slices at the bottom of the dish. Sprinkle the sausages over bread. Lay the tomatoes over it. Sprinkle top with cheese. Beat the eggs and then pour over top of bread slices.

2.   Drizzle vinegar and maple syrup over eggs. Flavor with Italian seasoning, salt, and pepper, then sprinkle some more cheese on top. Place the baking dish in the air fryer basket that should be preheated at

320 Fahrenheit and cooked for 10-minutes. Remove from air fryer and add a spot of mayonnaise and serve.

NUTRITION: Calories: 232 Total Fat: 7.4g Carbs: 6.3g Protein: 14.2g

9 Breakfast Muffins

Servings: 1 Cooking Time: 5 Minutes

1 medium egg
¼ cup heavy cream
1 slice cooked bacon (cured, pan-fried, cooked)
1 oz cheddar cheese
Salt and black pepper (to taste)

Direction:
1. Preheat the oven to 350°F.
2. In a bowl, mix the eggs with the cream, salt and pepper.
3. Spread into muffin tins and fill the cups half full.
4. Place 1 slice of bacon into each muffin hole and half ounce of cheese on top of each muffin.
5. Bake for around 15-20 minutes or until slightly browned.
6. Add another ½ oz of cheese onto each muffin and broil until the cheese is slightly browned.
7. Serve!

NUTRITION: Calories: 150 cal., 11g fat, 7g protein, 2g carbs

10 Baked Mini Quiche

Preparation Time: 10 minutes | Cooking Time: 15 minutes | Servings: 2

2 eggs
1 large yellow onion, diced
1 ¾ cups whole wheat flour
1 ½ cups spinach, chopped
¾ cup cottage cheese
Salt and black pepper to taste
2 tablespoons olive oil
¾ cup butter
¼ cup milk

1.   Preheat the air fryer to 355 Fahrenheit. Add the flour, butter, salt, and milk to the bowl and knead the dough until smooth and refrigerate for 15-minutes. Abode a frying pan over medium heat and add the oil to it. When the oil is heated, add the onions into the pan and sauté them. Improve spinach to pan and cook until it wilts.

2.   Drain excess moisture from spinach. Whisk the eggs together and add cheese to bowl and mix. Proceeds the dough out of the fridge and divide into 8 equal parts. Roll the dough into a round that will fit into the bottom of quiche mound. Place the rolled dough into molds. Place the spinach filling over dough.

3.   Place molds into air fryer basket and place basket inside of air fryer and cook for 15-minutes. Remove quiche from molds and serve warm or cold.

NUTRITION: Calories: 262 Total Fat: 8.2g Carbs: 7.3g Protein: 9.5g

11 Peanut Butter & Banana Breakfast Sandwich

Preparation Time: 10 minutes | Cooking Time: 6 minutes | Servings: 1

2 slices of whole wheat bread
1 teaspoon of sugar-free maple syrup
1 sliced banana
2 tablespoons of peanut butter

1.   Evenly coat both sides of the slices of bread with peanut butter. Add the sliced banana and drizzle with some sugar-free maple syrup.
2.   Heat in the air fryer to 330 Fahrenheit for 6 minutes. Serve warm.

NUTRITION: Calories: 211 Total Fat: 8.2g Carbs: 6.3g Protein: 11.2g

12 Egg and Avocado Breakfast Burrito

Preparation Time: 10 minutes | Cooking Time: 3 to 5 minutes | Servings: 4

2 hard-boiled egg whites, chopped
1 hard-boiled egg, chopped
1 avocado, peeled, pitted, and chopped
1 red bell pepper, chopped
3 tablespoons low-sodium salsa, plus additional for serving (optional)
1 (1.2-ounce / 34-g) slice low-sodium, low-fat American cheese, torn into pieces
4 low-sodium whole-wheat flour tortillas

1.   In a medium bowl, thoroughly mix the egg whites, egg, avocado, red bell pepper, salsa, and cheese.
2.   Place the tortillas on a work surface and evenly divide the filling among them. Fold in the edges and roll up. Secure the burritos with toothpicks if necessary.
3.   Put the burritos in the air fryer basket. Air fry at 390°F (199°C) for 3 to 5 minutes, or until the burritos are light golden brown and crisp. Serve with more salsa (if using).

NUTRITION: Calories: 205 Fat: 8g Protein: 9g Carbs: 27g Fiber: 3g Sugar: 1g Sodium: 109mg

Lunch

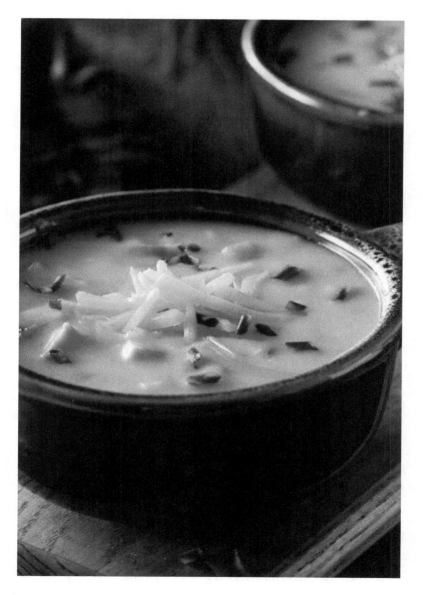

13 Beef Zoodle Stew

Prep time: 15 minutes, cook time; 1 hour 25 minutes,
Serves: 6

1 lb. beef stew meat
4 large zucchinis, spiralize
3 celery stalks, diced
3 carrots, peeled and diced
½ red onion, diced
What you'll need from store cupboard
14oz. can tomatoes, diced
4 cup low-sodium beef broth
2 cloves garlic, diced fine
1-2 bay leaves
3 tbsp. Worcestershire sauce
2 tbsp. olive oil
1 tsp thyme
½ tsp cayenne pepper
¼ tsp red pepper flakes
Salt and pepper, to taste
Freshly chopped parsley, to garnish

1.   Heat oil in a large saucepan over medium heat.
Add beef and cook until brown on all sides. Remove
from pan and set aside.
2.   Add the garlic to the pan and cook 30 seconds.
Then stir in onion and red pepper flakes. Cook 1 minute

and add the celery and carrots. Sweat the vegetables for 2 minutes, stirring occasionally.

3.   Add the beef back to the pan with the Worcestershire, thyme, and cayenne pepper and stir. Season with salt and pepper to taste. Add the broth, tomatoes, and bay leaves and bring to a boil.

4.   Reduce heat, cover and let simmer 40 minutes. Remove the cover and cook 35 minutes more or until stew thickens.

5.   Divide the zucchini noodles evenly among four bowls. Ladle stew evenly over zucchini and let set for a few minutes to cook the zucchini. Top with fresh parsley and serve.

NUTRITION: Calories 225 Total Carbs 13g Net Carbs 10g Protein 29g Fat 6g Sugar 8g Fiber 3g

14 Beer Cheese & Chicken Soup

Prep time: 15 minutes, cook time; 5 hours 30 minutes, Serves: 6-8

6 slices bacon, cut into 1 inch pieces
1 lb. chicken breast, cut into bite size pieces
2 cup half-and-half
1 cup cheddar cheese, grated
1 cup light beer
4 tbsp. margarine
What you'll need from store cupboard
1 cup low sodium chicken broth
¼ cup flour
2 tsp garlic powder
1 tsp cayenne pepper
1 tsp smoked paprika
1 tsp salt
1 tsp black pepper, coarsely ground
1 tsp Worcestershire sauce

1.   Cook bacon in a medium skillet, over med-high heat until almost crisp. Remove with a slotted spoon and add to crock pot.

2.   Add chicken to the skillet and cook until no longer pink. Add it to the bacon along with the broth,

beer, and Worcestershire. Cover and cook on low 4 hours.

3.   Melt margarine in a small saucepan over medium heat. Add flour and spices and whisk until smooth. Whisk in half-n-half and continue stirring until thoroughly combined. Stir into chicken mixture in crock pot.

4.   Add the cheese and stir well. Cook another 60-90 minutes or until cheese has completely melted and soup has thickened. Serve.

NUTRITION: Calories 453 Total Carbs 9g Protein 32g Fat 30g Sugar 0g Fiber 0g

15 Chili Chicken Wings

Preparation Time: 10 minutes, Cooking Time: 1 hour 10 minutes Servings: 4

2 lbs chicken wings
1/8 tsp. paprika
1/2 cup coconut flour
1/4 tsp. garlic powder
1/4 tsp. chili powder

Direction:
1. Preheat the oven to 400 F/ 200 C.
2. In a mixing bowl, add all ingredients except chicken wings and mix well.
3. Add chicken wings to the bowl mixture and coat well and place on a baking tray.
4. Bake in preheated oven for 55-60 minutes.
5. Serve and enjoy.

NUTRITION: Calories 440 Fat 17.1 g, Carbs 1.3 g, Sugar 0.2 g, Protein 65.9 g, Cholesterol 202 mg

16 Garlic Chicken Wings

Preparation Time: 10 minutes | Cooking Time: 55 minutes | Servings: 6

12 chicken wings
2 garlic clove, minced
3 tbsp. ghee
1/2 tsp. turmeric
2 tsp. cumin seeds

1. Preheat the oven to 425 F/ 215 C.
2. In a large bowl, mix together 1 teaspoon cumin, 1 tbsp. ghee, turmeric, pepper, and salt.
3. Add chicken wings to the bowl and toss well.
4. Spread chicken wings on a baking tray and bake in preheated oven for 30 minutes.
5. Turn chicken wings to another side and bake for 8 minutes more.
6. Meanwhile, heat remaining ghee in a pan over medium heat.
7. Add garlic and cumin to the pan and cook for a minute.
8. Remove pan from heat and set aside.
9. Remove chicken wings from oven and drizzle with ghee mixture/
10. Bake chicken wings 5 minutes more.
11. Serve and enjoy.

NUTRITION: Calories 378 Fat 27.9 g, Carbs 11.4 g, Sugar 0 g, Protein 19.7 g, Cholesterol 94 mg

17 Spinach Cheese Pie

Preparation Time: 10 minutes, Cooking Time: 40 minutes Servings: 8

6 eggs, lightly beaten
2 boxes frozen spinach, chopped
2 cup cheddar cheese, shredded
15 oz. cottage cheese
tsp. salt

Direction:
1. Preheat the oven to 375 F/ 190 C.
2. Spray an 8*8-inch baking dish with cooking spray and set aside.
3. In a mixing bowl, combine together spinach, eggs, cheddar cheese, cottage cheese, pepper, and salt.
4. Pour spinach mixture into the prepared baking dish and bake in preheated oven for 10 minutes.
5. Serve and enjoy.

NUTRITION: Calories 229 Fat 14 g, Carbs. 5.4 g, Sugar 0.9 g, Protein 21 g, Cholesterol 157 mg

18 Tasty Harissa Chicken

Preparation Time: 10 minutes, Cooking Time: 4 hours 10 minutes Servings: 4

lb. chicken breasts, skinless and boneless
1/2 tsp. ground cumin
1 cup harissa sauce
1/4 tsp. garlic powder
1/2 tsp. kosher salt

1. Season chicken with garlic powder, cumin, and salt.
2. Place chicken to the slow cooker.
3. Pour harissa sauce over the chicken.
4. Cover slow cooker with lid and cook on low for 4 hours.
5. Remove chicken from slow cooker and shred using a fork.
6. Return shredded chicken to the slow cooker and stir well.
7. Serve and enjoy.

NUTRITION: Calories 232 Fat 9.7 g, Carbs 1.3 g, Sugar 0.1 g, Protein 32.9 g, Cholesterol 101 mg

19 Festive Season Stuffed Tenderloin

Preparation Time: 10 minutes | Cooking Time: 45 minutes | Serving: 8 (1/8 of recipe serving)

4 teaspoons of olive oil, divided
2 minced shallots
1-8 ounce package sliced cremini mushrooms
3 minced garlic cloves, divided
1 tablespoon fresh thyme, chopped (add extra for garnish)
1 1/2 teaspoons fresh parsley, chopped (add extra for garnish)
1/4 cup dry sherry (or you can use red wine vinegar)
32 to 40 ounces beef tenderloin
1/2 cup bread crumbs, fresh whole wheat
1 teaspoon salt
1/2 teaspoon of black pepper

1.   Preheat your oven to 425degreesF.
2.   Heat 2 tablespoons oil over medium heat and cook shallots for 5 minutes or until tender. Add mushrooms and stir-cook until it softens (about 8 minutes).

3.   Stir in the garlic and herbs and cook for a minute more before adding the dry sherry. Reduce the sherry by half then remove and let it cool.

4.   Cut the beef lengthwise resembling butterfly wings. Cover with plastic and pound using a mallet until ½-inch thick.

5.   Stir in breadcrumbs in your mushroom mixture before spreading evenly onto the beef. Leave a 1-inch space around the edge.

6.   Roll the beef jellyroll style and secure with kitchen string at one-inch interval. Place the rolled meat on a rack inside a shallow roasting pan.

7.   Combine remaining ingredients and rub over the beef.

8.   Roast beef for 35-40 minutes for medium rare or according to your desired doneness.

9.   Let it cool 15-20 minutes with loosely tented foil before carving.

10.   Serve with extra thyme and parsley.

NUTRITION: Calories: 195 |Carbohydrates: 5 g |Fiber: 1 g |Fats: 9 g |Sodium: 381 mg |Protein: 21 g

20 Roasted Pork with Currant Sauce

Preparation Time: 10 minutes | Cooking Time: 1 hour | Serving: 6 (4 oz. serving)

1 boneless pork loin roast (2 pounds)
Marinade:
1-1/2 cups orange juice
1/4 cup lemon juice
2 teaspoons minced fresh gingerroot
1 teaspoon minced garlic
1 teaspoon dried oregano
1 teaspoon ground cinnamon
1/2 teaspoon ground coriander
1 small onion, sliced
Currant Sauce:
1 shallot, chopped
1 teaspoon minced garlic
1 tablespoon butter
1 tablespoon all-purpose _our
1/2 cup reduced-sodium chicken broth
1/2 cup red currant jelly

1.   Follow Steps 1 and 2 for Grilled Lamb Chops. Reserve 1 cup of the marinade.

2. Bake 1 hour at 350degreesF or until inserted kitchen thermometer reads 160degrees. Let it cool for 10 minutes before slicing. Set aside.

3. Sauté shallots and garlic in butter for a minute. Sprinkle flour and stir until blended. Gradually add the remaining ingredients and bring to a boil. Stir-cook for 2 minutes or until thick.

4. Serve with pork.

NUTRITION: Calories: 307 |Carbohydrates: 26 g |Fiber: 0 g |Fats: 9 g |Sodium: 115 mg |Protein: 30 g

21 Spicy Beef Sloppy Joes

Preparation Time: 20 minutes | Cooking Time: 8 hours | Servings: 12

Lean ground beef – 2 lb.
Lower-sodium salsa – 2 ½ cups
Coarsely chopped fresh mushrooms – 3 cups
Shredded carrots – 1 ¼ cups
Finely chopped red and green sweet peppers – 1 ¼ cups
No-salt added tomato paste – ½ (6-oz.) can
Garlic – 4 cloves, minced
Dried basil – 1 tsp. crushed
Salt – ¾ tsp.
Dried oregano – ½ tsp. crushed
Cayenne pepper – ¼ tsp.
Whole wheat hamburger buns – 12, split and toasted

1.   Cook ground beef in a skillet until browned. Drain off fat.
2.   In a slow cooker, add the meat and combine the next 10 ingredients (through cayenne pepper).
3.   Cover and cook on low for 8 to 10 hours or on high for 4 to 5 hours.
4.   Spoon ½-cup of the meat mixture onto each bun.
5.   Serve.

NUTRITION: Calories: 278 Fat: 8g Carb: 29g Protein: 20g

22 Skirt Steak With Asian Peanut Sauce

Prep Time: 10 minutes | Cooking Time: 15 Minutes | Servings: 4

⅓ cup light coconut milk
teaspoon curry powder
teaspoon coriander powder
1 teaspoon reduced-sodium soy sauce
1¼ pound skirt steak Cooking spray
½ cup Asian Peanut Sauce

1. In a large bowl, whisk together the coconut milk, curry powder, coriander powder, and soy sauce.
2. Add the steak and turn to coat.
3. Cover the bowl and refrigerate for at least 30 minutes and no longer than 24 hours.
4. Preheat the barbecue or coat a grill pan with cooking spray and place the steak over medium-high heat.
5. Grill the meat until it reaches an internal temperature of 145°F, about 3 minutes per side.
6. Remove the steak from the grill and let it rest for 5 minutes. Slice the steak into 5-ounce pieces and serve each with 2 tablespoons of the Asian Peanut Sauce.

7. REFRIGERATE: Store the cooled steak in a reseal able container for up to 1 week. Reheat each piece in the microwave for 1 minute.

NUTRITION: Calories: 361 Fat: 22g Saturated Fat: 7g Protein: 36g Total Carbs: 8g Fiber: 2g Sodium: 349mg

Dinner

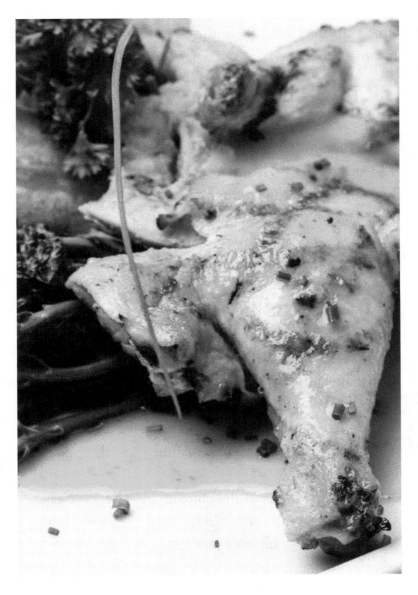

23 Greek Chicken Stuffed Peppers

Preparation time: 5 minutes | Cooking time: 30 minutes | Serves 4

2 large red bell peppers
2 teaspoons extra-virgin olive oil, divided
½ cup uncooked brown rice or quinoa
4 (4-ounce / 113-g) boneless, skinless chicken breasts
¼ teaspoon garlic powder
¼ teaspoon onion powder
⅛ teaspoon dried thyme
½ teaspoon dried oregano
½ cup crumbled feta

1.   Cut the bell peppers in half and remove the seeds.
2.   In a large skillet, heat 1 teaspoon of olive oil over low heat. When hot, place the bell pepper halves cut-side up in the skillet. Cover and cook for 20 minutes.
3.   Cook the rice according to the package instructions.
4.   Meanwhile, cut the chicken into 1-inch pieces.
5.   In a medium skillet, heat the remaining 1 teaspoon of olive oil over medium-low heat. When hot, add the chicken.

6.   Season the chicken with the garlic powder, onion powder, thyme, and oregano.

7.   Cook for 5 minutes, stirring occasionally, until cooked through.

8.   In a large bowl, combine the cooked rice and chicken. Scoop one-quarter of the chicken and rice mixture into each pepper half, cover, and cook for 10 minutes over low heat.

9.   Top each pepper half with 2 tablespoons of crumbled feta.

NUTRITION: calories: 288 | fat: 10g | protein: 32g | carbs: 20g | sugars: 4g | fiber: 4g | sodium: 267mg

24 Creole Chicken

Preparation time: 15 minutes | Cooking time: 25 minutes | Serves 2

2 chicken breast halves, boneless and skinless
1 cup cauliflower rice, cooked
⅓ cup green bell pepper, julienned
¼ cup celery, diced
¼ cup onion, diced
14½ ounces (411 g) stewed tomatoes, diced
1 teaspoon sunflower oil
1 teaspoon chili powder
½ teaspoon thyme
⅛ teaspoon pepper

1.   Heat oil in a small skillet over medium heat. Add chicken and cook 5 to 6 minutes per side or cooked through. Transfer to plate and keep warm.
2.   Add the pepper, celery, onion, tomatoes, and seasonings. Bring to a boil. Reduce heat, cover, and simmer 10 minutes or until vegetables start to soften.
3.   Add chicken back to pan to heat through. Serve over cauliflower rice.

NUTRITION: calories: 361 | fat: 14g | protein: 45g | carbs: 14g | fiber: 4g | sugars: 8g | sodium: 335mg

25 Cashew Chicken

Preparation time: 10 minutes | Cooking time: 10 minutes | Serves 4

1 pound skinless boneless chicken breast, cut in cubes
½ onion, sliced
2 tablespoons green onion, diced
½ teaspoon fresh ginger, peeled and grated
1 cup whole blanched cashews, toasted
1 clove garlic, diced fine
4 tablespoons oil
2 tablespoons dark soy sauce
2 tablespoons hoisin sauce
2 tablespoons water
2 teaspoons cornstarch
2 teaspoons dry sherry
1 teaspoon Splenda
1 teaspoon sesame seed oil

1.   Place chicken in a large bowl and add cornstarch, sherry, and ginger. Stir until well mixed.
2.   In a small bowl, whisk together soy sauce, hoisin, Splenda, and water stirring until smooth.
3.   Heat the oil in a wok or a large skillet over high heat. Add garlic and onion and cook, stirring until garlic sizzles, about 30 seconds.

4.   Stir in chicken and cook, stirring frequently, until chicken is almost done, about 2 minutes.

5.   Reduce heat to medium and stir in sauce mixture. Continue cooking and stirring until everything is blended together. Add cashews and cook 30 seconds.

6.   Drizzle with sesame oil, and cook another 30 seconds, stirring constantly. Serve immediately garnished with green onions.

NUTRITION: calories: 484 | fat: 32g | protein: 33g | carbs: 19g | fiber: 2g | sugars: 6g | sodium: 447mg

26 Citrus Chicken Thighs

Preparation time: 15 minutes | Cooking time: 30 minutes | Serves 4

1 tablespoon grated fresh ginger
Sea salt, to taste
4 chicken thighs, bone-in, skinless
1 tablespoon extra-virgin olive oil
Juice and zest of ½ orange
Juice and zest of ½ lemon
1 tablespoon low-sodium soy sauce
Pinch red pepper flakes, to taste
2 tablespoons honey
1 tablespoon chopped fresh cilantro

1.   In a large bowl, combine the ginger and salt. Dunk the chicken thighs and toss to coat well.
2.   Heat the olive oil in a nonstick skillet over medium-high heat until shimmering.
3.   Add the chicken thighs and cook for 10 minutes or until well browned. Flip halfway through the cooking time.
4.   Meanwhile, combine the orange juice and zest, lemon juice and zest, soy sauce, red pepper flakes, and honey. Stir to mix well.

5.   Pour the mixture in the skillet. Reduce the heat to low, then cover and braise for 20 minutes. Add tablespoons of water if too dry.

6.   Serve the chicken thighs garnished with cilantro.

NUTRITION: calories: 114 | fat: 5g | protein: 9g | carbs: 9g | fiber: 0g | sugars: 9g | sodium: 287mg

27 Turkey Meatball and Vegetable Kabobs

Prep time: 50 minutes | Cook time: 20 minutes | Serves 6

20 ounces lean ground turkey (93% fat-free)
2 egg whites
2 tablespoons grated Parmesan cheese
2 cloves garlic, minced
½ teaspoon salt, or to taste
¼ teaspoon ground black pepper
1 tablespoon olive oil
8 ounces fresh cremini mushrooms, cut in half to make 12 pieces
24 cherry tomatoes
1 medium onion, cut into 12 pieces
¼ cup balsamic vinegar

Special Equipment:
12 bamboo skewers, soaked in water for at least 30 minutes

1. Mix the ground turkey, egg whites, Parmesan, garlic, salt, and pepper in a large bowl. Stir to combine well.

2. Shape the mixture into 12 meatballs and place on a baking sheet. Refrigerate for at least 30 minutes.

3. Preheat the oven to 375°F (190°C). Grease another baking sheet with 1 tablespoon of olive oil.

4. Remove the meatballs from the refrigerator. Run the bamboo skewers through 2 meatballs, 1 mushroom, 2 cherry tomatoes, and 1 onion piece alternatively.

5. Arrange the kabobs on the greased baking sheet and brush with balsamic vinegar.

6. Grill in the preheated oven for 20 minutes or until an instant-read thermometer inserted in the middle of the meatballs reads at least 165°F (74°C). Flip the kabobs halfway through the cooking time.

7. Allow the kabobs to cool for 10 minutes, then serve warm.

NUTRITION: calories: 200 | fat: 8.0g | protein: 22.0g | carbs: 7.0g | fiber: 1.0g | sugar: 4.0g | sodium: 120mg

28 Mexican Turkey Sliders

Prep time: 15 minutes | Cook time: 6 minutes | Serves 7

1 pound lean ground turkey
1 tablespoon chili powder
½ teaspoon garlic powder
¼ teaspoon ground black pepper
7 mini whole-wheat hamburger buns
7 tomato slices
3½ slices reduced-fat pepper Jack cheese, cut in half
½ mashed avocado

1.   Preheat the grill to high heat.
2.   Combine the ground turkey, chili powder, garlic powder, and black pepper in a large bow. Stir to mix well.
3.   Divide and shape the mixture into 7 patties, then arrange the patties on the preheated grill grates.
4.   Grill for 6 minutes or until well browned. Flip the patties halfway through.
5.   Assemble the patties with buns, tomato slices, cheese slices, and mashed avocado to make the sliders, then serve immediately.

NUTRITION: calories: 225 | fat: 9.0g | protein: 17.0g | carbs: 21.0g | fiber: 4.0g | sugar: 6.0g | sodium: 230mg

29 Arroz Con Pollo

Prep time: 10 minutes | Cook time: 25 minutes | Serves 4

1 onion, diced
1 red pepper, diced
2 cup chicken breast, cooked and cubed
1 cup cauliflower, grated
1 cup peas, thaw
2 tablespoons cilantro, diced
½ teaspoon lemon zest
14½ ounces (411 g) low sodium chicken broth
¼ cup black olives, sliced
¼ cup sherry
1 clove garlic, diced
2 teaspoons olive oil
¼ teaspoon salt
¼ teaspoon cayenne pepper

1.   Heat oil in a large skillet over medium-high heat. Add pepper, onion and garlic and cook 1 minute. Add the cauliflower and cook, stirring frequently, until light brown, 4 to 5 minutes.

2.   Stir in broth, sherry, zest and seasonings. Bring to a boil. Reduce heat, cover and simmer 15 minutes.

3.   Stir in the chicken, peas and olives. Cover and simmer another 3 to 6 minutes or until heated through. Serve garnished with cilantro.

NUTRITION: calories: 162 | fat: 5.0g | protein: 14.2g | carbs: 13.1g | fiber: 4.2g | sugar: 5.1g | sodium: 307mg

30 Scallion Sandwich

Preparation Time: 10 minutes | Cooking Time: 10 minutes | Servings: 1

2 slices wheat bread
2 teaspoons butter, low fat
2 scallions, sliced thinly
1 tablespoon of parmesan cheese, grated
3/4 cup of cheddar cheese, reduced fat, grated

1.   Preheat the Air fryer to 356 degrees.
2.   Spread butter on a slice of bread. Place inside the cooking basket with the butter side facing down.
3.   Place cheese and scallions on top. Spread the rest of the butter on the other slice of bread Put it on top of the sandwich and sprinkle with parmesan cheese.
4.   Cook for 10 minutes.

NUTRITION: Calorie: 154Carbohydrate: 9g Fat: 2.5g Protein: 8.6g Fiber: 2.4g

31 Lean Lamb and Turkey Meatballs with Yogurt

Preparation Time: 10 minutes | Cooking Time: 8 minutes | Servings: 4

2 egg white
4 ounces ground lean turkey
2 pound of ground lean lamb
1 teaspoon each of cayenne pepper, ground coriander, red chili paste, salt, and ground cumin
2 garlic cloves, minced
1/2 tablespoons parsley, chopped
1/4 cup of olive oil
1 tablespoon mint, chopped,
For the yogurt
2 tablespoons of buttermilk
garlic clove, minced
1/4 cup mint, chopped
1/2 cup of Greek yogurt, non-fat
Salt to taste

1.	Set the Air Fryer to 390 degrees.
2.	Mix all the ingredients for the meatballs in a bowl. Roll and mold them into golf-size round pieces. Arrange in the cooking basket. Cook for 8 minutes.

3.   While waiting, combine all the ingredients for the mint yogurt in a bowl. Mix well.

4.   Serve the meatballs with the mint yogurt. Top with olives and fresh mint.

NUTRITION: Calorie: 154 Carbohydrate: 9g Fat: 2.5g Protein: 8.6g Fiber: 2.4g

32 Air Fried Section and Tomato

Preparation Time: 10 minutes | Cooking Time: 5 minutes | Servings: 2

Aubergine, sliced thickly into 4 disks
Tomato, sliced into 2 thick disks
2 tsp. feta cheese, reduced fat
2 fresh basil leaves, minced
2 balls, small buffalo mozzarella, reduced fat, roughly torn
Pinch of salt
Pinch of black pepper

1.   Preheat Air Fryer to 330 degrees F.
2.   Spray small amount of oil into the Air fryer basket. Fry aubergine slices for 5 minutes or until golden brown on both sides. Transfer to a plate.
3.   Fry tomato slices in batches for 5 minutes or until seared on both sides.
4.   To serve, stack salad starting with an aborigine base, buffalo mozzarella, basil leaves, tomato slice, and 1/2-teaspoon feta cheese.
5.   Top of with another slice of aborigine and 1/2 tsp. feta cheese. Serve.

NUTRITION: Calorie: 140.3 Carbohydrate: 26.6 Fat: 3.4g Protein: 4.2g Fiber: 7.3g

Sides

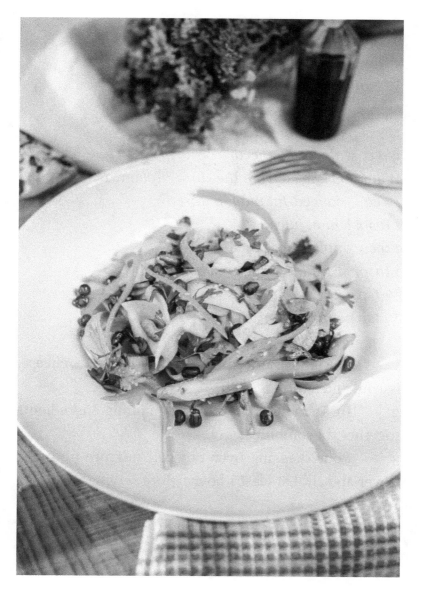

33 Broccoli & Bacon Salad

Prep time: 10 minutes, Serves: 4

2 cups broccoli, separated into florets
4 slices bacon, chopped and cooked crisp
½ cup cheddar cheese, cubed
¼ cup low-fat Greek yogurt
1/8 cup red onion, diced fine
1/8 cup almonds, sliced
What you'll need from the store cupboard
¼ cup reduced-fat mayonnaise
1 tbsp. lemon juice
1 tbsp. apple cider vinegar
1 tbsp. granulated sugar substitute
¼ tsp salt
¼ tsp pepper

1.   In a large bowl, combine broccoli, onion, cheese, bacon, and almonds.
2.   In a small bowl, whisk remaining Ingredients together till combined.
3.   Pour dressing over broccoli mixture and stir. Cover and chill at least 1 hour before serving.

NUTRITION: Calories 217 Total Carbs 12g Net Carbs 10g Protein 11g Fat 14g Sugar 6g Fiber 2g

34 Chopped Veggie Salad

Total time: 15 minutes, Serves: 4

1 cucumber, chopped
1 pint cherry tomatoes, cut in half
3 radishes, chopped
1 yellow bell pepper chopped
½ cup fresh parsley, chopped
What you'll need from store cupboard:
3 tbsp. lemon juice
1 tbsp. olive oil
Salt to taste

1.   Place all Ingredients in a large bowl and toss to combine. Serve immediately, or cover and chill until ready to serve.

NUTRITION: Calories 70 Total Carbs 9g Net Carbs 7g Protein 2g Fat 4g Sugar 5g Fiber 2g

35 Pickled Cucumber & Onion Salad

Total time: 10 minutes, Serves: 2

½ cucumber, peeled and sliced
¼ cup red onion, sliced thin
What you'll need from store cupboard:
1 tbsp. olive oil
1 tbsp. white vinegar
1 tsp dill

1.   Place all Ingredients in a medium bowl and toss to combine. Serve.

NUTRITION: Calories 79 Total Carbs 4g Net Carbs 3g Protein 1g Fat 7g Sugar 2g Fiber 1g

36 Mashed Butternut Squash

Preparation time: 5   minutes Cooking Time: 25 minutes Servings: 6

3 pounds whole butternut squash (about 2 medium)
2 tablespoons olive oil
Salt and pepper

1. Preheat the oven to 400F and line a baking sheet with parchment.
2. Cut the squash in half and remove the seeds.
3. Cut the squash into cubes and toss with oil then spread on the baking sheet.
4. Roast for 25 minutes until tender then place in a food processor.
5. Blend smooth then season with salt and pepper to taste.

NUTRITION: Calories 90, Total Fat 4.8g, Total Carbs 12.3g, Protein 1.1g, Sugar 2.3g, Fiber 2.1g, Sodium 4mg

37 Cilantro Lime Quinoa

Preparation time: 5 minutes | Cooking Time: 25 minutes | Servings: 6

cup uncooked quinoa
tablespoon olive oil
medium yellow onion, diced
2 cloves minced garlic
1 (4-ounce) can diced green chiles, drained
1/2 cups fat-free chicken broth
¾ cup fresh chopped cilantro
1/2 cup sliced green onion
2 tablespoons lime juice
Salt and pepper

1. Rinse the quinoa thoroughly in cool water using a fine mesh sieve.
2. Heat the oil in a large saucepan over medium heat.
3. Add the onion and sauté for 2 minutes then stir in the chile and garlic.
4. Cook for 1 minute then stir in the quinoa and chicken broth.
5. Bring to a boil then reduce heat and simmer, covered, until the quinoa absorbs the liquid – about 20 to 25 minutes.
6. Remove from heat then stir in the cilantro, green onions, and lime juice.

7. Season with salt and pepper to taste and serve hot.

NUTRITION: Calories 150, Total Fat 4.1g, Total Carbs 22.5g, Protein 6g, Sugar 1.7g, Fiber 2.7g, Sodium 179mg

38 Oven-Roasted Veggies

Preparation time: 5 minutes Cooking |Time: 25 minutes | Servings: 6

pound cauliflower florets
1/2 pound broccoli florets
large yellow onion, cut into chunks
1 large red pepper, cored and chopped
2 medium carrots, peeled and sliced
2 tablespoons olive oil
2 tablespoons apple cider vinegar
Salt and pepper

1. Preheat the oven to 425F and line a large rimmed baking sheet with parchment.
2. Spread the veggies on the baking sheet and drizzle with oil and vinegar.
3. Toss well and season with salt and pepper.
4. Spread the veggies in a single layer then roast for 20 to 25 minutes, stirring every 10 minutes, until tender.
5. Adjust seasoning to taste and serve hot.

NUTRITION: Calories 100, Total Fat 5g, Total Carbs 12.4g, Protein 3.2g, Sugar 5.5g, Fiber 4.2g, Sodium 51mg

39 Vegetable Rice Pilaf

Preparation time: 5 minutes Cooking | Time: 25 minutes | Servings: 6

tablespoon olive oil
1/2 medium yellow onion, diced
cup uncooked long-grain brown rice
2 cloves minced garlic
1/2 teaspoon dried basil
Salt and pepper
2 cups fat-free chicken broth
cup frozen mixed veggies

1. Heat the oil in a large skillet over medium heat.
2. Add the onion and sauté for 3 minutes until translucent.
3. Stir in the rice and cook until lightly toasted.
4. Add the garlic, basil, salt, and pepper then stir to combined.
5. Stir in the chicken broth then bring to a boil.
6. Reduce heat and simmer, covered, for 10 minutes.
7. Stir in the frozen veggies then cover and cook for another 10 minutes until heated through. Serve hot.

NUTRITION: Calories 90, Total Fat 2.7g, Total Carbs 12.6g, Protein 3.9g, Sugar 1.5g, Fiber 2.2g, Sodium 143mg

40 Curry Roasted Cauliflower Florets

Preparation time: 5 minutes| Cooking Time: 25 minutes | Servings: 6

8 cups cauliflower florets
2 tablespoons olive oil
1 teaspoon curry powder
1/2 teaspoon garlic powder
Salt and pepper

1. Preheat the oven to 425F and line a baking sheet with foil.
2. Toss the cauliflower with the olive oil and spread on the baking sheet.
3. Sprinkle with curry powder, garlic powder, salt, and pepper.
4. Roast for 25 minutes or until just tender. Serve hot.

NUTRITION: Calories 75, Total Fat 4.9g, Total Carbs 7.4g, Protein 2.7g, Sugar 3.3g, Fiber 3.5g, Sodium 40mg

41 Baked Veggies Combo

Preparation Time: 15 minutes | Cooking Time: 40 minutes | Servings: 8

large zucchinis, sliced
large yellow squash, sliced
cups fresh broccoli florets
1-pound fresh asparagus, trimmed
garlic cloves, minced
1 tablespoon fresh rosemary, minced
1 tablespoon fresh thyme, minced
½ teaspoon ground cumin
½ teaspoon red pepper flakes, crushed
¼ teaspoon cayenne pepper
tablespoons olive oil
Salt, as required

1. Preheat the oven to 400 degrees F. Line 2 large baking sheets with aluminum foil. In a large bowl, add all ingredients and toss to coat well.
2. Divide the vegetables mixture onto prepared baking sheets and spread in a single layer.
3. Roast for about 35-40 minutes. Remove from oven and serve.
4. Meal Prep Tip:
5. Remove from oven and set the veggies aside to cool completely.

6. Transfer the veggie mixture into 8 containers and refrigerate for 2-3 days.
7. Reheat in microwave before serving.

NUTRITION: Calories 77, Total Fat 4 g, Total Carbs 9.4 g, Sugar 3.8 g, Fiber 3.8 g, Sodium 45 mg, Potassium 554 mg, Protein 3.8 g

42 Mixed Veggie Salad

Preparation Time: 20 minutes Servings: 8

For Dressing:
1/3 cup olive oil
½ cup fresh lemon juice
tablespoon fresh ginger, grated
teaspoons mustard 4-6 drops liquid stevia
¼ teaspoon salt
For Salad:
avocados, peeled, pitted and chopped
tablespoons fresh lemon juice
cups fresh baby spinach, torn
cups small broccoli florets
cup red cabbage, shredded
cup purple cabbage, shredded
large carrots, peeled and grated
small orange bell pepper, seeded and sliced into matchsticks
small yellow bell pepper, seeded and sliced into matchsticks
½ cup fresh parsley leaves, chopped
cup walnuts, chopped

1. For dressing: in a food processor, add all ingredients and pulse until well combined. In a

large bowl, add the avocado slices and drizzle with lemon juice.

2. Add the remaining vegetables and mix. Place the dressing and toss to coat well.

3. Serve immediately.

4. Meal Prep Tip:

5. Transfer dressing into a small jar and refrigerate for 1 day. In 8 containers, divide avocado and remaining vegetables.

6. Refrigerate for 1 day. Before serving, drizzle each portion with dressing and serve.

NUTRITION: Calories 314 Total Fat 28.1 g Total Carbs 14.1 g Sugar 4.3g Fiber 6.9 g Sodium 113 mg Potassium 642 mg Protein 6.8 g

Desserts

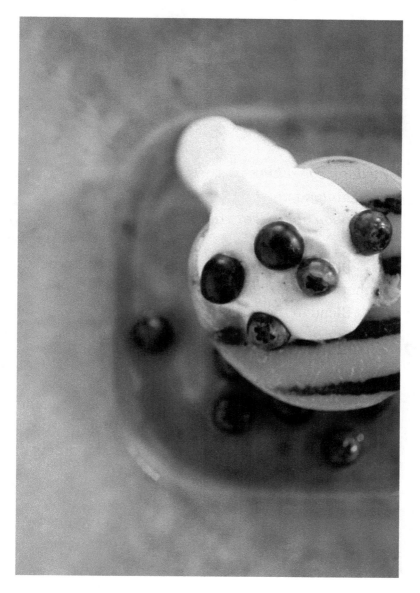

43 Peach and Almond Meal Fritters

Preparation time: 15 minutes | Cooking time: 15 minutes | Serves 7

4 ripe bananas, peeled
2 cups chopped peaches
1 medium egg
2 medium egg whites
¾ cup almond meal
¼ teaspoon almond extract

1.   In a large bowl, mash the bananas and peaches together with a fork or potato masher.
2.   Blend in the egg and egg whites.
3.   Stir in the almond meal and almond extract.
4.   Working in batches, place ¼-cup portions of the batter into the basket of an air fryer.
5.   Set the air fryer to 390°F (199°C), close, and cook for 12 minutes.
6.   Once cooking is complete, transfer the fritters to a plate. Repeat until no batter remains.

NUTRITION: calories: 164 | fat: 7g | protein: 6g | carbs: 22g | sugars: 12g | fiber: 4g | sodium: 23mg

44 Tapioca Berry Parfaits

Preparation time: 10 minutes | Cooking time: 6 minutes | Serves 4

2 cups unsweetened almond milk
½ cup small pearl tapioca, rinsed and still wet
1 teaspoon almond extract
1 tablespoon pure maple syrup
2 cups berries
¼ cup slivered almonds

1.   Pour the almond milk into the electric pressure cooker. Stir in the tapioca and almond extract.
2.   Close and lock the lid of the pressure cooker. Set the valve to sealing.
3.   Cook on High pressure for 6 minutes.
4.   When the cooking is complete, hit Cancel. Allow the pressure to release naturally for 10 minutes, then quick release any remaining pressure.
5.   Once the pin drops, unlock and remove the lid. Remove the pot to a cooling rack.
6.   Stir in the maple syrup and let the mixture cool for about an hour.
7.   In small glasses, create several layers of tapioca, berries, and almonds. Refrigerate for 1 hour.
8.   Serve chilled.

NUTRITION: (6 tablespoons tapioca, ½ cup berries, and 1 tablespoon almonds) calories: 174 | fat: 5g | protein: 3g | carbs: 32g | sugars: 11g | fiber: 3g | sodium: 77mg

45 Blackberry Yogurt Ice Pops

Preparation time: 10 minutes | Cooking time: 0 minutes | Serves 4

12 ounces (340 g) plain Greek yogurt
1 cup blackberries
Pinch nutmeg
¼ cup milk
2 (1-gram) packets stevia

1. In a blender, combine all of the ingredients. Blend until smooth.
2. Pour the mixture into 4 ice pop molds. Freeze for 6 hours before serving.

NUTRITION: calories: 75 | fat: 6g | protein: 9g | carbs: 9g | sugars: 5g | fiber: 2g | sodium: 7mg

46 Chocolate Almond Butter Fudge

Preparation time: 10 minutes | Cooking time: 0 minutes | Makes 9 pieces

2 ounces unsweetened baking chocolate
½ cup almond butter
1 can full-fat coconut milk, refrigerated overnight, thickened cream only
1 teaspoon vanilla extract
4 packets stevia (or to taste)

1.   Line a 9-inch square baking pan with parchment paper.
2.   In a small saucepan over medium-low heat, heat the chocolate and almond butter, stirring constantly, until both are melted. Cool slightly.
3.   In a medium bowl, combine the melted chocolate mixture with the cream from the coconut milk, vanilla, and stevia. Blend until smooth. Taste and adjust sweetness as desired.
4.   Pour the mixture into the prepared pan, spreading with a spatula to smooth. Refrigerate for 3 hours. Cut into squares.

NUTRITION: (1 piece) calories: 200 | fat: 20g | protein: 4g | carbs: 6g | sugars: 2g | fiber: 2g | sodium: 8mg

47 Cream Cheese Pound Cake

Prep time: 10 minutes | Cook time: 35 minutes | Serves 14

4 eggs
3.25 ounces (92 g) cream cheese, soft
4 tablespoons butter, soft
1¼ cup almond flour
¾ cup Splenda
1 teaspoon baking powder
1 teaspoon of vanilla
¼ teaspoon salt
Butter flavored cooking spray

1.   Heat oven to 350°F (180°C). Spray a loaf pan with cooking spray.
2.   In a medium bowl, combine flour, baking powder, and salt.
3.   In a large bowl, beat butter and Splenda until light and fluffy. And cream cheese and vanilla and beat well.
4.   Add the eggs, one at a time, beating after each one. Stir in the dry until thoroughly combined.
5.   Pour into prepared pan and bake for 30 to 40 minutes or cake passes the toothpick test. Let cool 10 minutes in the pan, then invert onto serving plate. Slice and serve.

NUTRITION: calories: 203 | fat: 13.0g | protein: 5.0g | carbs: 15.1g | fiber: 1.0g | sugar: 13.1g | sodium: 84mg

48 Gingerbread Soufflés

Prep time: 15 minutes | Cook time: 25 minutes | Serves 10

6 eggs, separated
1 cup skim milk
1 cup fat free whipped topping
2 tablespoons butter, soft
½ cup Splenda
⅓ cup molasses
¼ cup flour
2 teaspoons pumpkin pie spice
2 teaspoons vanilla
1 teaspoon ginger
¼ teaspoon salt
⅛ teaspoon cream of tartar
Butter flavored cooking spray

1.   Heat oven to 350°F (180°C). Spray 10 ramekins with cooking spray and sprinkle with Splenda to coat, shaking out excess. Place on a large baking sheet.

2.   In a large saucepan, over medium heat, whisk together milk, Splenda, flour and salt until smooth. Bring to a boil, whisking constantly. Pour into a large bowl and whisk in molasses, butter, vanilla, and spices. Let cool 15 minutes.

3.   Once spiced mixture has cooled, whisk in egg yolks.

4.   In a large bowl, beat egg whites and cream of tartar on high speed until stiff peaks form. Fold into spiced mixture, a third at a time, until blended completely. Spoon into ramekins.

5.   Bake for 25 minutes until puffed and set. Serve immediately with a dollop of whipped topping.

NUTRITION: calories: 171 | fat: 5.0g | protein: 4.0g | carbs: 24.1g | fiber: 0g | sugar: 18.1g | sodium: 289mg

49 Mini Bread Puddings

Prep time: 5 minutes | Cook time: 35 minutes | Serves 12

6 slices cinnamon bread, cut into cubes
1¼ cup skim milk
½ cup egg substitute
1 tablespoon margarine, melted
⅓ cup Splenda
1 teaspoon vanilla
⅛ teaspoon salt
⅛ teaspoon nutmeg

1.   Heat oven to 350°F (180°C). Line 12 medium-size muffin cups with paper baking cups.
2.   In a large bowl, stir together milk, egg substitute, Splenda, vanilla, salt and nutmeg until combined. Add bread cubes and stir until moistened. Let rest 15 minutes.
3.   Spoon evenly into prepared baking cups. Drizzle margarine evenly over the tops. Bake for 30 to 35 minutes or until puffed and golden brown. Remove from oven and let cool completely.

NUTRITION: calories: 106 | fat: 2.0g | protein: 4.0g | carbs: 16.1g | fiber: 1.0g | sugar: 9.1g | sodium: 118mg

50 Mini Key Lime Tarts

Prep time: 5 minutes | Cook time: 10 minutes | Serves 8

4 sheets phyllo dough
¾ cup skim milk
¾ cup fat-free whipped topping, thawed
½ cup egg substitute
½ cup fat free sour cream
6 tablespoons fresh lime juice
2 tablespoons cornstarch
½ cup Splenda
Butter-flavored cooking spray

1.	In a medium saucepan, combine milk, juice, and cornstarch. Cook, stirring, over medium heat 2 to 3 minutes or until thickened. Remove from heat.

2.	Add egg substitute and whisk 30 seconds to allow it to cook. Stir in sour cream and Splenda. Cover and chill until completely cool.

3.	Heat oven to 350°F (180°C). Spray 8 muffin cups with cooking spray.

4.	Lay 1 sheet of the phyllo on a cutting board and lightly spray it with cooking spray. Repeat this with the remaining sheets so they are stacked on top of each other.

5.   Cut the phyllo into 8 squares and gently place them in the prepared muffin cups, pressing firmly on the bottom and sides. Bake for 8 to 10 minutes or until golden brown. Remove them from the pan and let cool.

6.   To serve: spoon the lime mixture evenly into the 8 cups and top with whipped topping. Garnish with fresh lime slices if desired.

NUTRITION: calories: 83 | fat: 1.0g | protein: 3.0g | carbs: 13.1g | fiber: 1.0g | sugar: 10.1g | sodium: 111mg

51 Grilled Peach and Coconut Yogurt Bowls

Preparation Time: 5 Minutes | Cooking Time: 10 Minutes | Servings: 4

2 Peaches, halved and pitted
½ cup plain nonfat Greek yogurt
1 teaspoon pure vanilla extract
¼ cup unsweetened dried coconut flakes
2 tablespoons unsalted pistachios, shelled and broken into pieces

1. Preheat the broiler to high. Arrange the rack in the closest position to the broiler.
2. In a shallow pan, arrange the peach halves, cut-side up. Broil for 6 to 8 minutes until browned, tender, and hot.
3. In a small bowl, mix the yogurt and vanilla.
4. Spoon the yogurt into the cavity of each peach half.
5. Sprinkle one tablespoon of coconut flakes and 1½ teaspoons of pistachios over each peach half. Serve warm.

NUTRITION: Calories: 102 Total Fat: 5g Protein: 5g Carbohydrates: 11g

52 Chocolate Peanut Butter Freezer Bites

Preparation Time: 8 Minutes | Cooking Time: 0 Minutes |Servings: 32

1 cup coconut oil, melted
¼ cup cocoa powder
¼ cup honey
¼ cup natural peanut butter

1.   Pour the melted coconut oil into a medium bowl. Whisk in the cocoa powder, honey, and peanut butter.
2.   Transfer the mixture to ice cube trays in portions of about 1½ teaspoons each.
3.   Freeze for 2 hours or until ready to serve.

NUTRITION: Calories: 80 Fat: 8g Protein: 1g Carbohydrates: 3g

53 Dark Chocolate Almond Butter cups

Preparation Time: 55 Minutes | Cooking Time: 0 Minutes | Servings: 12

½ cup natural almond butter
1 tablespoon pure maple syrup
1 cup dark chocolate chips
1 tablespoon coconut oil

1.   Line a 12-cup muffin tin with cupcake liners.
2.   In a medium bowl, mix the almond butter and maple syrup. If necessary, heat in the microwave to soften slightly.
3.   Spoon about two teaspoons of the almond butter mixture into each muffin cup and press down to fill.
4.   In a double boiler or the microwave, melt the chocolate chips. Stir in the coconut oil, and mix well to incorporate.
5.   Drop one tablespoon of chocolate on top of each almond buttercup.
6.   Freeze for at least 30 minutes to set. Thaw for 10 minutes before serving.

NUTRITION: Calories: 101 Total Fat: 8g Protein: 3g Carbohydrates: 6g

54 Carrot Cake Bites

Preparation Time: 14 Minutes | Cooking Time: 0 Minutes | Servings: 20

½ cup old-fashioned oats
2 medium carrots, chopped
6 dates, pitted
½ cup chopped walnuts
½ cup coconut flour
2 tablespoons hemp seeds
2 teaspoons pure maple syrup
1 teaspoon ground cinnamon
½ teaspoon ground nutmeg

1.   In a blender jar, combine the oats and carrots, and process until finely ground. Transfer to a bowl.
2.   Add the dates and walnuts to the blender and process until coarsely chopped. Return the oat-carrot mixture to the blender and add the coconut flour, hemp seeds, maple syrup, cinnamon, and nutmeg. Process until well mixed.
3.   Using your hands, shape the dough into balls about the size of a tablespoon.
4.   Store in the refrigerator in an airtight container for up to 1 week.

NUTRITION: Calories: 68 Total Fat: 3g Protein: 2g Carbohydrates: 10g

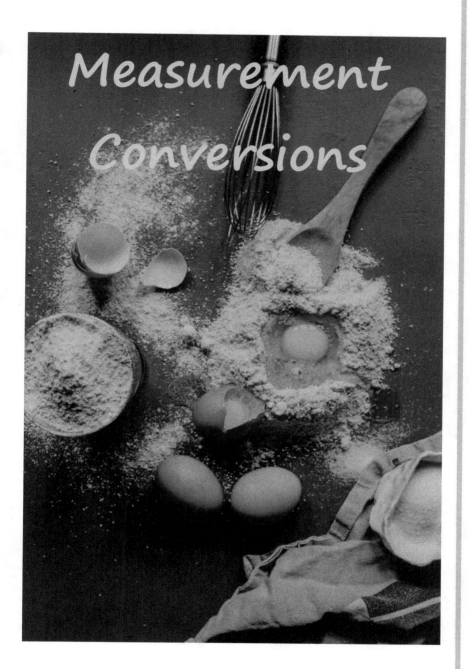

Measurement Conversions

VOLUME EQUIVALENTS (LIQUID)

US STANDARD	US STANDARD (OUNCES)	METRIC (APPROXIMATE)
2 tablespoons	1 fl. oz.	30 mL
¼ cup	2 fl. oz.	60 mL
½ cup	4 fl. oz.	120 mL
1 cup	8 fl. oz.	240 mL
1 ½ cups	12 fl. oz.	355 mL
2 cups or 1 pint	16 fl. oz.	475 mL
4 cups or 1 quart	32 fl. oz.	1 L
1 gallon	128 fl. oz.	4 L

US STANDARD	METRIC (APPROXIMATE)
⅛ teaspoon	0.5 mL
¼ teaspoon	1 mL
½ teaspoon	2 mL
¾ teaspoon	4 mL
1 teaspoon	5 mL
1 tablespoon	15 mL
¼ cup	59 mL
⅓ cup	79 mL
½ cup	118 mL
⅔ cup	156 mL
¾ cup	177 mL
1 cup	235 mL
2 cups or 1 pint	475 mL
3 cups	700 mL
4 cups or 1 quart	1 L

OVEN TEMPERATURES

FAHRENHEIT	CELSIUS (APPROXIMATE)
250°F	120°C
300°F	150°C
325°F	165°C
350°F	180°C
375°F	190°C
400°F	200°C
425°F	220°C
450°F	230°C

WEIGHT EQUIVALENTS

US STANDARD	METRIC (APPROXIMATE)
½ ounce	15 g
1 ounce	30 g
2 ounces	60 g
4 ounces	115 g
8 ounces	225 g
12 ounces	340 g
16 ounces or 1 pound	455 g